One Step Med

One Step Med

General Medical Information
Record Keeping Manual

CHINETHA M. CRENSHAW

Ordering Information:

For orders and inquiries, please contact:
1-888-404-1388
www.goldtouchpress.com
book.orders@goldtouchpress.com

Printed in the United States of America

Name: ____

Mailing Address: ____

____

____

Birth Place: (city, state, country) ____

____

____

Employer: ____

Occupation: ____

Date Retired: ____

Marital Status: (married, single, divorced, or widowed)

____

If you are a veteran please complete this information:

Service number: ____

____

Branch: ____

____

Date enlisted:____

____

Rank:____

____

Name of war: ____

____

Date Discharged: ____

____

Location of original discharge papers: _______________________________________

____

Date of Birth: ____

Blood Type: ____

Social History:

____
____
____
____
____
____
____
____
____
____

Do you have a Medical Power of Attorney? Yes ____________ No ____________

Emergency Contact Information: ______________________________________

____
____
____
____

Primary Insurance Information: _______________________________________

____
____
____
____

Secondary Insurance Information: _____________________________________

____
____
____
____

          CHINETHA M. CRENSHAW

Allergies:

____
____
____
____
____
____
____
____
____
____

Blood Pressure, Blood Sugar, Height, Weight, BMI, Glucose Level and Cholesterol:________

____
____
____
____
____
____
____
____
____
____

Diseases:

____
____
____
____
____
____
____
____
____
____

Allergies:

____

____

____

____

____

____

____

____

Blood Pressure, Blood Sugar, Height, Weight, BMI, Glucose Level and Cholesterol:_______

____

____

____

____

____

____

____

____

____

____

Diseases:

____

____

____

____

____

____

____

____

____

____

Allergies:

____
____
____
____
____
____
____
____
____

Blood Pressure, Blood Sugar, Height, Weight, BMI, Glucose Level and Cholesterol:________

____
____
____
____
____
____
____
____
____
____

Diseases:

____
____
____
____
____
____
____
____
____
____

Worker's Compensation, Disability and Social Security Information:

Injury Date: ____

Claim # ____

____

Diagnosis code(s), Approval Dates, and Form Expiration Dates:

____

____

____

____

____

____

____

____

____

____

MCO Information and Case Manager:

____

____

____

____

____

____

____

____

Worker's Compensation Physician(s), Referrals and Contact Information:

____

____

____

____

____

____

____

____

                    CHINETHA M. CRENSHAW

Worker's Compensation, Disability and Social Security Information:

Injury Date: ____

Claim # ____

____

Diagnosis code(s), Approval Dates, and Form Expiration Dates:

____

____

____

____

____

____

____

____

____

MCO Information and Case Manager:

____

____

____

____

____

____

____

____

Worker's Compensation Physician(s), Referrals and Contact Information:

____

____

____

____

____

____

____

____

____

Worker's Compensation, Disability and Social Security Information:

Injury Date: ____

Claim # ____

____

Diagnosis code(s), Approval Dates, and Form Expiration Dates:

____

____

____

____

____

____

____

____

____

MCO Information and Case Manager:

____

____

____

____

____

____

____

Worker's Compensation Physician(s), Referrals and Contact Information:

____

____

____

____

____

____

____

                    CHINETHA M. CRENSHAW

Worker's Compensation, Disability and Social Security Information:

Injury Date: ____

Claim # ____

____

Diagnosis code(s), Approval Dates, and Form Expiration Dates:

____

____

____

____

____

____

____

____

____

____

MCO Information and Case Manager:

____

____

____

____

____

____

____

____

____

Worker's Compensation Physician(s), Referrals and Contact Information:

____

____

____

____

____

____

____

____

____

Please list Counselor, Case Manager, Social Worker, Therapist or Psychiatrist, etc:

Name(s): ____

____

____

____

Contact Information: ____

Address: ____

____

____

____

Phone number(s): ____

____

____

____

Referral Contact Information: ____

____

____

____

Diagnosis and Recommended Medication(s): ____

____

____

____

____

Details of Session, including recommended treatment with start and completion date(s):

____

____

____

____

____

Please list Counselor, Case Manager, Social Worker, Therapist or Psychiatrist, etc:

Name(s): ____

____

____

____

Contact Information: ____

Address: ____

____

____

____

Phone number(s): ____

____

____

____

Referral Contact Information: ____

____

____

____

Diagnosis and Recommended Medication(s): __________________________________

____

____

____

____

____

Details of Session, including recommended treatment with start and completion date(s):

____

____

____

____

____

Important Family History (note important medical history of each family member including mother, father, brother(s), sister(s), children, etc.):

CHINETHA M. CRENSHAW

Important Family History (note important medical history of each family member including mother, father, brother(s), sister(s), children, etc.):

Important Family History (note important medical history of each family member including mother, father, brother(s), sister(s), children, etc.):

CHINETHA M. CRENSHAW

Important Family History (note important medical history of each family member including mother, father, brother(s), sister(s), children, etc.):

Important Family History (note important medical history of each family member including mother, father, brother(s), sister(s), children, etc.):

Important Personal History (note important medical history):

____
____
____
____
____
____
____
____
____
____
____
____
____
____
____
____
____
____
____
____
____
____
____
____
____
____
____
____
____
____

Important Personal History (note important medical history):

                    CHINETHA M. CRENSHAW

Important Personal History (note important medical history):

Important Personal History (note important medical history):

Important Personal History (note important medical history):

Medical Procedures (past or present):

Diagnosis: ____

____

____

Treatment: ____

____

____

Surgery: Y/N

Date(s): ____

Hospital: ____

Medication(s)-dosage and purpose of: ______________________________

____

____

____

____

____

____

____

____

____

Comments on treating physician(s), recommended treatment, and prescribed medications:

____

____

____

____

____

____

____

____

____

____

____

____

     CHINETHA M. CRENSHAW

Medical Procedures (past or present):

Diagnosis: ____

____

____

Treatment: ____

____

____

Surgery: Y/N

Date(s): ____
Hospital: ____

Medication(s)-dosage and purpose of: _______________________________

____

____

____

____

____

____

____

____

Comments on treating physician(s), recommended treatment, and prescribed medications:

____

____

____

____

____

____

____

____

____

____

____

____

Medical Procedures (past or present):

Diagnosis: ____

____

____

Treatment: ____

____

____

Surgery: Y/N

Date(s): ____

Hospital: ____

Medication(s)-dosage and purpose of: ___________________________________

____

____

____

____

____

____

____

____

Comments on treating physician(s), recommended treatment, and prescribed medications:

____

____

____

____

____

____

____

____

____

____

____

____

     CHINETHA M. CRENSHAW

Medical Procedures (past or present):

Diagnosis: ____

____

____

Treatment: ____

____

____

Surgery: Y/N

Date(s): ____
Hospital: ____

Medication(s)-dosage and purpose of: ______________________________

____

____

____

____

____

____

____

____

Comments on treating physician(s), recommended treatment, and prescribed medications:

____

____

____

____

____

____

____

____

____

____

____

____

Medical Procedures (past or present):

Diagnosis: ____

____

____

Treatment: ____

____

____

Surgery: Y/N

Date(s): ____
Hospital: ____

Medication(s)-dosage and purpose of: _______________________

____

____

____

____

____

____

____

____

Comments on treating physician(s), recommended treatment, and prescribed medications:

____

____

____

____

____

____

____

____

____

____

____

Infections (list past or present, dates of, and suggested treatment):

____

____

____

____

____

____

____

____

____

____

____

____

____

Test Dates, Exam Dates, and Results:

____

____

____

____

____

____

____

____

____

____

____

____

____

Infections (list past or present, dates of, and suggested treatment):

____
____
____
____
____
____
____
____
____
____
____
____
____
____

Test Dates, Exam Dates, and Results:

____
____
____
____
____
____
____
____
____
____
____
____
____
____
____
____

　　　　CHINETHA M. CRENSHAW

Infections (list past or present, dates of, and suggested treatment):

Test Dates, Exam Dates, and Results:

Infections (list past or present, dates of, and suggested treatment):

____

____

____

____

____

____

____

____

____

____

____

____

____

Test Dates, Exam Dates, and Results:

____

____

____

____

____

____

____

____

____

____

____

____

____

____

     CHINETHA M. CRENSHAW

Infections (list past or present, dates of, and suggested treatment):

____
____
____
____
____
____
____
____
____
____
____
____
____
____
____

Test Dates, Exam Dates, and Results:

____
____
____
____
____
____
____
____
____
____
____
____
____
____

X-Rays, Cat Scans, MRIs, EMGs, ECG or EKG, etc. (diagnosis and discovery):

CHINETHA M. CRENSHAW

X-Rays, Cat Scans, MRIs, EMGs, ECG or EKG, etc. (diagnosis and discovery):

X-Rays, Cat Scans, MRIs, EMGs, ECG or EKG, etc. (diagnosis and discovery):

X-Rays, Cat Scans, MRIs, EMGs, ECG or EKG, etc. (diagnosis and discovery):

X-Rays, Cat Scans, MRIs, EMGs, ECG or EKG, etc. (diagnosis and discovery):

Ultra Sound, OBGYN (Pap), Colonoscopy, Prostate or Testicular-related Test and Results:

Ultra Sound, OBGYN (Pap), Colonoscopy, Prostate or Testicular-related Test and Results:

Ultra Sound, OBGYN (Pap), Colonoscopy, Prostate or Testicular-related Test and Results:

Ultra Sound, OBGYN (Pap), Colonoscopy, Prostate or Testicular-related Test and Results:

Ultra Sound, OBGYN (Pap), Colonoscopy, Prostate or Testicular-related Test and Results:

Dental Procedures, Eye Exams, and Hearing Tests (list dates and results):

CHINETHA M. CRENSHAW

Dental Procedures, Eye Exams, and Hearing Tests (list dates and results):

Dental Procedures, Eye Exams, and Hearing Tests (list dates and results):

CHINETHA M. CRENSHAW

Dental Procedures, Eye Exams, and Hearing Tests (list dates and results):

Dental Procedures, Eye Exams, and Hearing Tests (list dates and results):

    CHINETHA M. CRENSHAW

IMMUNIZATIONS, HEALTH SCREENING AND VACCINE: (note year received; never received; or unsure)

Shingles ____

Covid-19 ____

Tetanus Vaccine ____

Flu Vaccine ____

Pneumonia In j ____

Hepatitis B ____

other ____

____

____

____

____

____

____

____

____

____

Pharmacy Name(s), Addresses, and Phone number(s):

____

____

____

____

____

____

____

____

____

____

____

____

____

____

IMMUNIZATIONS, HEALTH SCREENING AND VACCINE: (note year received; never received; or unsure)

Shingles ____

Covid-19 ____

Tetanus Vaccine ____

Flu Vaccine ____

Pneumonia In j ____

Hepatitis B ____

other ____

____

____

____

____

____

____

____

____

____

____

____

Pharmacy Name(s), Addresses, and Phone number(s):

____

____

____

____

____

____

____

____

____

____

____

____

____

____

____

____

 CHINETHA M. CRENSHAW

IMMUNIZATIONS, HEALTH SCREENING AND VACCINE: (note year received; never received; or unsure)

Shingles ____

Covid-19 ____

Tetanus Vaccine ____

Flu Vaccine ____

Pneumonia In j ____

Hepatitis B ____

other ____

____

____

____

____

____

____

____

____

____

Pharmacy Name(s), Addresses, and Phone number(s):

____

____

____

____

____

____

____

____

____

____

____

____

____

____

IMMUNIZATIONS, HEALTH SCREENING AND VACCINE: (note year received; never received; or unsure)

Shingles ____

Covid-19 ____

Tetanus Vaccine ____

Flu Vaccine ____

Pneumonia In j ____

Hepatitis B ____

other ____

____

____

____

____

____

____

____

____

____

____

Pharmacy Name(s), Addresses, and Phone number(s):

____

____

____

____

____

____

____

____

____

____

____

____

____

____

　　　　CHINETHA M. CRENSHAW

IMMUNIZATIONS, HEALTH SCREENING AND VACCINE: (note year received; never received; or unsure)

Shingles ____

Covid-19 ____

Tetanus Vaccine ____

Flu Vaccine ____

Pneumonia In j ____

Hepatitis B ____

other ____

____

____

____

____

____

____

____

____

____

Pharmacy Name(s), Addresses, and Phone number(s):

____

____

____

____

____

____

____

____

____

____

____

____

____

____

IMMUNIZATIONS, HEALTH SCREENING AND VACCINE: (note year received; never received; or unsure)

Shingles ____

Covid-19 ____

Tetanus Vaccine ____

Flu Vaccine ____

Pneumonia In j ____

Hepatitis B ____

other ____

____

____

____

____

____

____

____

____

____

____

Pharmacy Name(s), Addresses, and Phone number(s):

____

____

____

____

____

____

____

____

____

____

____

____

____

     CHINETHA M. CRENSHAW

IMMUNIZATIONS, HEALTH SCREENING AND VACCINE: (note year received; never received; or unsure)

Shingles ____

Covid-19 ____

Tetanus Vaccine ____

Flu Vaccine ____

Pneumonia In j ____

Hepatitis B ____

other ____

____

____

____

____

____

____

____

____

____

____

Pharmacy Name(s), Addresses, and Phone number(s):

____

____

____

____

____

____

____

____

____

____

____

____

____

____

____

IMMUNIZATIONS, HEALTH SCREENING AND VACCINE: (note year received; never received; or unsure)

Shingles ____

Covid-19 ____

Tetanus Vaccine ____

Flu Vaccine ____

Pneumonia In j ____

Hepatitis B ____

other ____

____

____

____

____

____

____

____

____

____

____

Pharmacy Name(s), Addresses, and Phone number(s):

____

____

____

____

____

____

____

____

____

____

____

____

____

____

____

   CHINETHA M. CRENSHAW

Important Medical To Do List continued (include appointments or procedures to schedule, prescriptions to request from physician, pick up or renew, and questions or concerns to ask physician or pharmacist):

Important Medical To Do List continued (include appointments or procedures to schedule, prescriptions to request from physician, pick up or renew, and questions or concerns to ask physician or pharmacist):

Important Medical To Do List continued (include appointments or procedures to schedule, prescriptions to request from physician, pick up or renew, and questions or concerns to ask physician or pharmacist):

Important Medical To Do List continued (include appointments or procedures to schedule, prescriptions to request from physician, pick up or renew, and questions or concerns to ask physician or pharmacist):

Important Medical To Do List continued (include appointments or procedures to schedule, prescriptions to request from physician, pick up or renew, and questions or concerns to ask physician or pharmacist):

Important Medical To Do List continued (include appointments or procedures to schedule, prescriptions to request from physician, pick up or renew, and questions or concerns to ask physician or pharmacist):

CHINETHA M. CRENSHAW

Medicines Used and Reactions (note reasons for use of drug with start and stop dates and list all past and current prescriptions, dosage and non-prescription drugs used):

Medicines Used and Reactions (note reasons for use of drug with start and stop dates and list all past and current prescriptions, dosage and non-prescription drugs used):

____

____

____

CHINETHA M. CRENSHAW

Medicines Used and Reactions (note reasons for use of drug with start and stop dates and list all past and current prescriptions, dosage and non-prescription drugs used):

Medicines Used and Reactions (note reasons for use of drug with start and stop dates and list all past and current prescriptions, dosage and non-prescription drugs used):

Medicines Used and Reactions (note reasons for use of drug with start and stop dates and list all past and current prescriptions, dosage and non-prescription drugs used):

Medicines Used and Reactions (note reasons for use of drug with start and stop dates and list all past and current prescriptions, dosage and non-prescription drugs used):

REVIEW OF SYSTEMS: Please keep a note of all symptoms you have had or are currently experiencing:

GENERAL

Fever
Chills
Night sweats
Weight loss/Weight gain
Depression
Fatigue
Trouble sleeping
Fainting/blackouts
Severe nervousness

SKIN

Dry skin
Rash or lesion
Itching
Easy bruising
Change in mole

EARS/NOSE/THROAT

Ear pain
Ringing in the ears
Difficulty hearing
Ear pressure
Nosebleeds
Drainage from the nose
Nasal congestion
Sneezing
Sore throat
Hoarseness
Difficulty swallowing
Sores in mouth

<u>EYES</u>
Glaucoma
Blurred vision
Double vision
Cataract

<u>RESPIRATORY</u>
Difficulty breathing/
Shortness of breath
Cough
Wheezing
Coughing up blood
Producing sputum (phlegm)

<u>CARDIOVASCULAR</u>
Chest pain, tightness or pressure
Shortness of breath with activities (working, walking, climbing stairs etc.)
Irregular or rapid heart beat (palpitations)
Leg swelling
Pain in legs when walking
Waking up at night with shortness of breath Shortness of breath when lying down

<u>GASTROINTESTINAL</u>
Loss of appetite or poor appetite
Vomiting
Nausea
Constipation
Diarrhea
Indigestion/heartburn
Ulcers
Stomach pain
Change in stools
Bright red blood in stools
Black/tarry stools

 CHINETHA M. CRENSHAW

<u>**REVIEW OF SYSTEMS continued:**</u>

Unable to control bowels
Gas
Vomiting blood
Bloating

<u>GENITOLURINARY</u>

Difficulty urinating
Urinating frequently, small amounts
Urinating frequently, normal or large amounts
Pain with urinating
Dribble urine
Blood in urine
Difficulty holding urine
Urinating at night (more than once each night)

<u>MUSKULOSKELETAL</u>

Joint pain
Joint stiffness
Low back pain
Neck pain
Muscle aches
Restless legs

<u>NEUROLOGY</u>

Dizziness
Headache
Lightheadedness
Memory loss/forgetfulness
Spinning sensation (vertigo)
Convulsions (seizures)
Tingling
Paralysis

<u>**REVIEW OF SYSTEMS continued:**</u>

<u>**ENDOCRINOLOGY**</u>
Diabetes
Thyroid disease
Increased appetite
Increased thirst
Unable to tolerate heat
Unable to tolerate cold
Excess facial hair or body hair
Change in head size

<u>**REVIEW OF SYSTEMS continued:**</u>

<u>**FOR WOMEN**</u>
Breast pain
Breast lump
Nipple discharge
Vaginal discharge (color or smell)
Pain with intercourse
Using birth control
Sexual problem
Previous sexually transmitted disease: gonorrhea, chlamydia, syphilis, herpes
Age period started
Date of last period
Duration of flow (days)
Pain with periods (minimal, moderate, severe)
Periods have stopped
Bleeding between periods
Irregular periods
Heavy periods
Bleeding after menopause
Hot flashes
Problems with contraceptive
of pregnancies

                    CHINETHA M. CRENSHAW

<u>**REVIEW OF SYSTEMS continued:**</u>

of miscarriages
of abortions
of live births Other

<u>**FOR MEN**</u>
Prostate problems
Sexual problems

<u>**REVIEW OF SYSTEMS continued:**</u>

Lump in testicle
Breast lump
Penis discharge
Sore on penis
Problems with contraceptive
Do you do a testicular self-exam?
Other

<u>**FOR CHILDREN**</u>
Constitutional (weight loss, low grade fever, fatigue)
Changes In Social Situation
Eyes (blurred or double vision, eye discharge)
Ear, Nose, Throat (nasal discharges, nose bleed, snoring, hearing loss, ringing in the ears)
Gastrointestinal (heartburn, nausea, vomiting, abdominal movements) Cardiac/Heart (chest pain, palpitations—to pulsate with unnatural rapidity, exercise intolerance)
Respiratory (cough, difficulty breathing)
Skeletal
Genitourinary (bed wetting, pain with urination, blood in urine. menstrual periods)
Skin (rashes)
Neurology/Muscular (changes in voice, choking, weakness, dizziness, numbness, changes in walking)
Endocrine (hot flashes, feeling cold, fatigue, excessive thirst, frequent urinating)
Hematology (pallor—unnatural paleness, recurrent fever)
Allergic/Immunologic—immunity from disease
Psychiatric/Behavioral (hallucinations, delusions, changes in mood)

Medical Concerns
(Review of Symptoms Notes)

Medical Concerns
(Review of Symptoms Notes)

Medical Concerns
(Review of Symptoms Notes)

Medical Concerns
(Review of Symptoms Notes)

Medical Concerns
(Review of Symptoms Notes)

Medical Concerns
(Review of Symptoms Notes)

Medical Concerns
(Review of Symptoms Notes)

Homegrown Remedies, Not to be forgotten:

Homegrown Remedies, Not to be forgotten:

Homegrown Remedies, Not to be forgotten:

Homegrown Remedies, Not to be forgotten:

CHINETHA M. CRENSHAW

Business Card Information

(Keep all current and past physician contact information)

NAME: ____

____

ADDRESS: ____

____

PHONE NUMBER(S): ____

EMAIL ADDRESS: ____

FAX: ____

SECRETARY or NAME OF OFFICE CONTACT: ____

____

NAME: ____

____

ADDRESS: ____

____

PHONE NUMBER(S): ____

EMAIL ADDRESS: ____

FAX: ____

SECRETARY or NAME OF OFFICE CONTACT: ____

____

QUICK NOTE: ____

____

____

Business Card Information

(Keep all current and past physician contact information)

NAME: ____

____

ADDRESS: ____

____

PHONE NUMBER(S): ____

EMAIL ADDRESS: ____

FAX: ____

SECRETARY or NAME OF OFFICE CONTACT: _______________________________

____

NAME: ____

____

ADDRESS: ____

____

PHONE NUMBER(S): ____

EMAIL ADDRESS: ____

FAX: ____

SECRETARY or NAME OF OFFICE CONTACT: _______________________________

____

QUICK NOTE: ____

____

____

Business Card Information

(Keep all current and past physician contact information)

NAME: ____

____

ADDRESS: ____

____

PHONE NUMBER(S): ____

EMAIL ADDRESS: ____

FAX: ____

SECRETARY or NAME OF OFFICE CONTACT: _______________________________

____

NAME: ____

____

ADDRESS: ____

____

PHONE NUMBER(S): ____

EMAIL ADDRESS: ____

FAX: ____

SECRETARY or NAME OF OFFICE CONTACT: _______________________________

____

QUICK NOTE: ____

____

____

Personal Notes

(Keep notes of opinion on: office visit, interaction with physician, feedback from physician, and if your visit was satisfactory or unsatisfactory with explanation)

Personal Notes

(Keep notes of opinion on: office visit, interaction with physician, feedback from physician, and if your visit was satisfactory or unsatisfactory with explanation)

Personal Notes

(Keep notes of opinion on: office visit, interaction with physician, feedback from physician, and if your visit was satisfactory or unsatisfactory with explanation)

Personal Notes

(Keep notes of opinion on: office visit, interaction with physician, feedback from physician, and if your visit was satisfactory or unsatisfactory with explanation)

Personal Notes

(Keep notes of opinion on: office visit, interaction with physician, feedback from physician, and if your visit was satisfactory or unsatisfactory with explanation)

CHINETHA M. CRENSHAW

Personal Notes

(Keep notes of opinion on: office visit, interaction with physician, feedback from physician, and if your visit was satisfactory or unsatisfactory with explanation)

Personal Notes

(Keep notes of opinion on: office visit, interaction with physician, feedback from physician, and if your visit was satisfactory or unsatisfactory with explanation)